YOU WILL SURVIVE MENOPAUSE

YOU WILL SURVIVE MENOPAUSE

Read Daily for Affirmation Book Series

Walter the Educator

Silent King Books

SILENT KING BOOKS

SKB

Copyright © 2024 by Walter the Educator

All rights reserved. No part of this book may be reproduced in any manner whatsoever without written permission except in the case of brief quotations embodied in critical articles and reviews.

First Printing, 2024

Disclaimer
This book is a literary work; poems are not about specific persons, locations, situations, and/or circumstances unless mentioned in a historical context. This book is for entertainment and informational purposes only. The author and publisher offer this information without warranties expressed or implied. No matter the grounds, neither the author nor the publisher will be accountable for any losses, injuries, or other damages caused by the reader's use of this book. The use of this book acknowledges an understanding and acceptance of this disclaimer.

Read this little poetry book daily and affirm that *You Will Survive Menopause*. I pray that you will survive menopause.

For where two or three are gathered together in my name, there am I in the midst of them – Matthew 18:20

Menopause, a chapter in life's endless book,

YOU WILL SURVIVE MENOPAUSE

A journey of rediscovery, a fresh outlook.

YOU WILL SURVIVE MENOPAUSE

No longer confined by society's chains,

YOU WILL SURVIVE MENOPAUSE

She finds freedom in her veins.

YOU WILL SURVIVE MENOPAUSE

"I will survive," she roars with delight,

YOU WILL SURVIVE MENOPAUSE

In the darkness of night, in the morning's bright light.

YOU WILL SURVIVE MENOPAUSE

With each step forward, she reclaims her might,

YOU WILL SURVIVE MENOPAUSE

A warrior of wisdom, shining ever so bright.

YOU WILL SURVIVE MENOPAUSE

The years unfold, a tapestry vast,

YOU WILL SURVIVE MENOPAUSE

Menopause, a passage, not meant to last.

YOU WILL SURVIVE MENOPAUSE

In the eyes of the woman, a flicker of dawn,

YOU WILL SURVIVE MENOPAUSE

A new day rises, and she carries on.

YOU WILL SURVIVE MENOPAUSE

Through tears and laughter, through loss and gain,

YOU WILL SURVIVE MENOPAUSE

She finds her rhythm, her own sweet refrain.

YOU WILL SURVIVE MENOPAUSE

Her story, a symphony, unique and grand,

YOU WILL SURVIVE MENOPAUSE

In the orchestra of life, she takes her stand.

YOU WILL SURVIVE MENOPAUSE

The echoes of time, a gentle reminder,

YOU WILL SURVIVE MENOPAUSE

Of the strength within, a spirit kinder.

YOU WILL SURVIVE MENOPAUSE

She walks with grace, with purpose anew,

YOU WILL SURVIVE MENOPAUSE

In the garden of life, where the flowers grew.

YOU WILL SURVIVE MENOPAUSE

Menopause, a journey, a transformative ride,

YOU WILL SURVIVE MENOPAUSE

In every challenge, a newfound pride.

YOU WILL SURVIVE MENOPAUSE

With resilience as her anchor, and hope as her guide,

YOU WILL SURVIVE MENOPAUSE

She navigates the waves, with love by her side.

YOU WILL SURVIVE MENOPAUSE

"I will survive," she proclaims with zest,

YOU WILL SURVIVE MENOPAUSE

In every heartbeat, in every breath.

YOU WILL SURVIVE MENOPAUSE

With courage unwavering, she faces the tide,

YOU WILL SURVIVE MENOPAUSE

A testament of strength, a woman's pride.

YOU WILL SURVIVE MENOPAUSE

In the heart of the storm, she finds her calm,

YOU WILL SURVIVE MENOPAUSE

In the cradle of change, a soothing balm.

YOU WILL SURVIVE MENOPAUSE

Her story unfolds, with each passing day,

YOU WILL SURVIVE MENOPAUSE

A masterpiece of life, in a glorious array.

YOU WILL SURVIVE MENOPAUSE

Menopause, a journey of strength and grace,

YOU WILL SURVIVE MENOPAUSE

In every challenge, a sacred space.

YOU WILL SURVIVE MENOPAUSE

Through the night's embrace, and the morning's rise,

YOU WILL SURVIVE MENOPAUSE

She discovers her power, her spirit's prize.

YOU WILL SURVIVE MENOPAUSE

With love in her heart, and fire in her soul,

YOU WILL SURVIVE MENOPAUSE

She navigates menopause, making herself whole.

YOU WILL SURVIVE MENOPAUSE

In the tapestry of life, she finds her place,

YOU WILL SURVIVE MENOPAUSE

A woman of wisdom, a beacon of grace.

YOU WILL SURVIVE MENOPAUSE

"I will survive," she declares with pride,

YOU WILL SURVIVE MENOPAUSE

In the ebb and flow, in the changing tide.

YOU WILL SURVIVE MENOPAUSE

Through the journey of menopause, she finds her stride,

YOU WILL SURVIVE MENOPAUSE

A warrior of light, forever by her side.

YOU WILL SURVIVE MENOPAUSE

ABOUT THE CREATOR

Walter the Educator is one of the pseudonyms for Walter Anderson. Formally educated in Chemistry, Business, and Education, he is an educator, an author, a diverse entrepreneur, and he is the son of a disabled war veteran. "Walter the Educator" shares his time between educating and creating. He holds interests and owns several creative projects that entertain, enlighten, enhance, and educate, hoping to inspire and motivate you.

> Follow, find new works, and stay up to date
> with Walter the Educator™
> at WaltertheEducator.com

www.ingramcontent.com/pod-product-compliance
Lightning Source LLC
La Vergne TN
LVHW052007060526
838201LV00059B/3886